The Ultimate Vegetarian Lunch Cooking Guide

Delicious Vegetarian Lunch Recipes For Everyone

Adam Denton

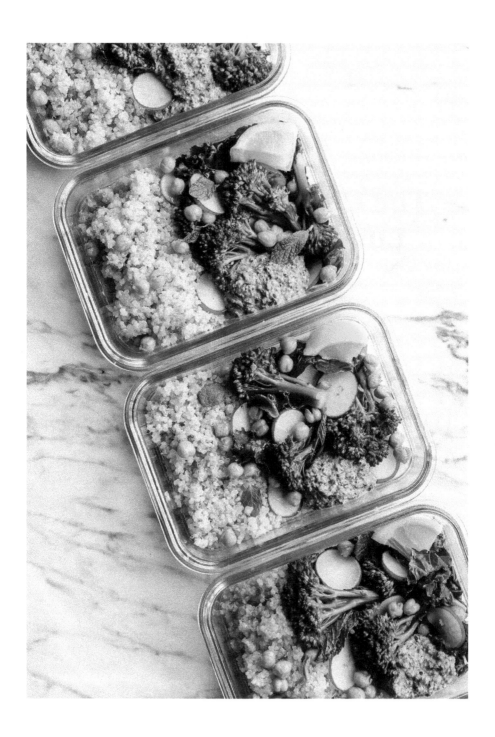

Table of contents

Chinese Roasted Button Mushrooms and Butternut Squash

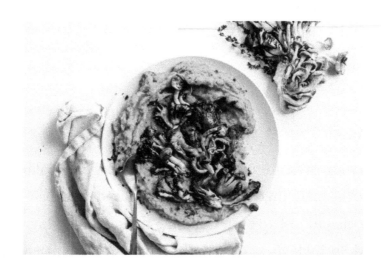

Ingredients

2 (15 ounce) cans button mushrooms, sliced and drained

1/2 butternut squash - peeled, seeded, and cut into 1-inch pieces

1 red onion, diced

2 large carrots, cut into 1 inch pieces

3 medium turnips, cut into 1-inch pieces

3 tablespoons sesame oil

Seasoning Ingredients

1 teaspoon salt

1/2 teaspoon ground black pepper

1 teaspoon onion powder

2 teaspoon garlic powder

1 teaspoon Sichuan peppercorns

1 teaspoon Chinese five-spice powder

Garnishing Ingredients

2 green onions, chopped (optional)

Directions:

Preheat your oven to 350 degrees F. Grease your baking pan. Combine the main Ingredients on the prepared sheet pan. Drizzle with the oil and toss to coat. Combine the seasoning Ingredients in a bowl Sprinkle them over the vegetables on the pan and toss to coat with seasonings. Bake in the oven for 25 minutes. Stir frequently until vegetables are soft and lightly browned and chickpeas are crisp, for about 20 to 25 minutes more. Season with more salt and black pepper to taste, top with the green onion before serving.

Roasted Button Mushrooms and Squash

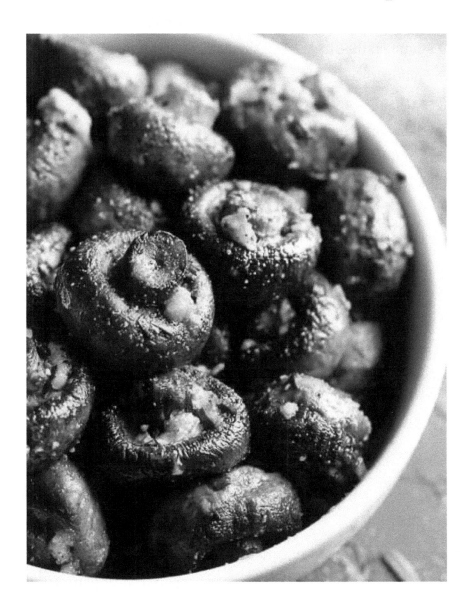

Ingredients

2 (15 ounce) cans button mushrooms, rinsed and drained

1/2 summer squash - peeled, seeded, and cut into 1-inch pieces

1 red onion, diced

2 large turnips, cut into 1 inch pieces

2 large parsnips, cut into 1 inch pieces

3 medium potatoes, cut into 1-inch pieces

3 tablespoons butter

Seasoning Ingredients

1 teaspoon salt

1/2 teaspoon ground black pepper

1 teaspoon onion powder

2 teaspoon garlic powder

1 teaspoon Herbs de Provence

Garnishing Ingredients

2 sprigs of thyme, chopped (optional)

Directions:

Preheat your oven to 350 degrees F. Grease your baking pan. Combine the main Ingredients on the prepared sheet pan. Drizzle with the melted butter or margarine and toss to coat. Combine the seasoning Ingredients in a bowl Sprinkle them over the vegetables on the pan and toss to coat with seasonings. Bake in the oven for 25 minutes. Stir frequently until vegetables are soft and lightly browned and chickpeas are crisp, for about 20 to 25 minutes more. Season with more salt and black pepper to taste, top with thyme before serving.

Roasted Turnips and Butternut Squash

Ingredients

3 medium tomatoes, cut into 1-inch pieces

1/2 butternut squash - peeled, seeded, and cut into 1-inch pieces

1 red onion, diced 1 turnip, peeled and cut into 1-inch cubes

2 large carrots, cut into 1 inch pieces

2 large kohlrabi, cut into 1 inch pieces

3 tablespoons extra virgin olive oil

Seasoning Ingredients

1 teaspoon salt

1/2 teaspoon ground black pepper

1 teaspoon onion powder

2 teaspoongarlic powder

1 teaspoon dried thyme

Garnishing Ingredients

2 sprigs fresh thyme, chopped (optional)

Directions:

Preheat your oven to 350 degrees F. Grease your baking pan. Combine the main Ingredients on the prepared sheet pan. Drizzle with the oil and toss to coat. Combine the seasoning Ingredients in a bowl Sprinkle them over the vegetables on the pan and toss to coat with seasonings. Bake in the oven for 25 minutes. Stir frequently until vegetables are soft and lightly browned and chickpeas are crisp, for about 20 to 25 minutes more. Season with more salt and black pepper to taste, top with the thyme before serving.

Roasted Tomatoes Rutabaga and Kohlrabi Main

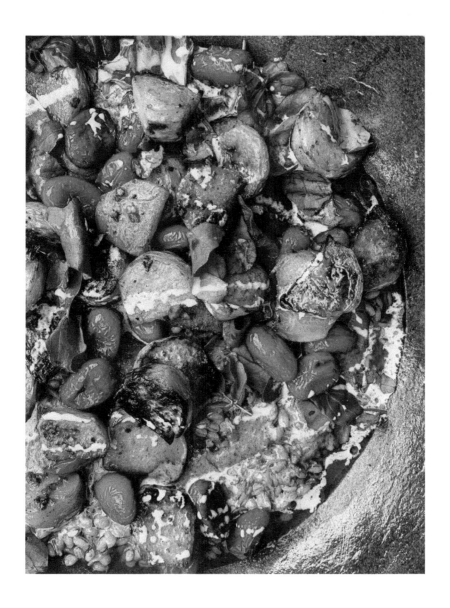

Ingredients

3 large tomatoes, cut into 1-inch pieces

3 red onion, diced 1 rutabaga, peeled and cut into 1-inch cubes

2 large carrots, cut into 1 inch pieces

3 medium kohlrabi, cut into 1-inch pieces

3 tablespoons extra virgin olive oil

Seasoning Ingredients

1 teaspoon salt

1/2 teaspoonground black pepper

1 teaspoon onion powder

2 teaspoongarlic powder

1 teaspoon Spanish paprika

1 teaspoon cumin

Garnishing Ingredients

2 sprigs parsley, chopped (optional)

Directions:

Preheat your oven to 350 degrees F. Grease your baking pan. Combine the main Ingredients on the prepared sheet pan. Drizzle with the oil and toss to coat. Combine the seasoning Ingredients in a bowl Sprinkle them over the vegetables on the pan and toss to coat with seasonings.

Bake in the oven for 25 minutes. Stir frequently until vegetables are soft, for about 20 to 25 minutes more. Season with more salt and black pepper to taste, top with the parsley before serving.

Roasted Butternut Squash Bean Sprouts and Broccoli

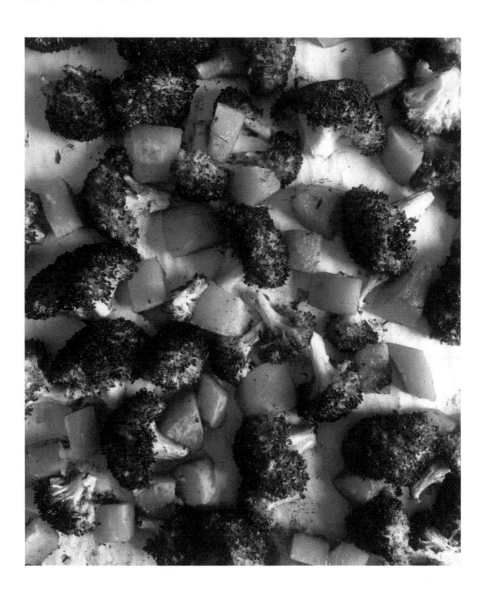

Ingredients

1 large broccoli, sliced

1 cup bean sprouts

1/2 butternut squash - peeled, seeded, and cut into 1-inch pieces

2 red onions, diced

2 large carrots, cut into 1 inch pieces

4 medium potatoes, cut into 1-inch pieces

3 tablespoons sesame oil

Seasoning Ingredients

1 teaspoon sea salt

1/2 teaspoonground black pepper

1 teaspoon onion powder

2 teaspoongarlic powder

1 teaspoon Sichuan peppercorns

Garnishing Ingredients

2 green onions, chopped (optional)

Directions:

Preheat your oven to 350 degrees F. Grease your baking pan. Combine the main Ingredients on the prepared sheet pan. Drizzle with the oil and toss to coat. Combine the seasoning Ingredients in a bowl Sprinkle them over the vegetables on the pan and toss to coat with seasonings. Bake in the oven for 25 minutes. Stir frequently until vegetables are soft and lightly browned and chickpeas are crisp, for about 20 to 25 minutes more. Season with more salt and black pepper to taste, top with the green onion before serving.

Roasted Brussel Sprouts and Brocccoli

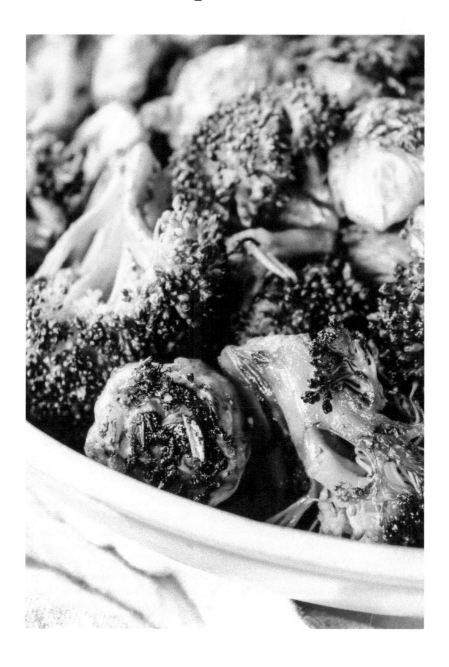

Ingredients

1 large broccoli, sliced

1 cup bean sprouts

1 red onion, diced

3 large kohlrabi, cut into 1 inch pieces

2 large carrots, cut into 1 inch pieces

3 medium potatoes, cut into 1-inch pieces

3 tablespoons extra virgin olive oil

<u>Seasoning Ingredients</u>

1 teaspoon salt

1/2 teaspoonground black pepper

1 teaspoon onion powder

2 teaspoongarlic powder

1 teaspoon ground fennel seeds

1 teaspoon dried rubbed sage

<u>Garnishing Ingredients</u>

2 green onions, chopped (optional)

Directions:

Preheat your oven to 350 degrees F. Grease your baking pan. Combine the main Ingredients on the prepared sheet pan. Drizzle with the oil and toss to coat. Combine the seasoning Ingredients in a bowl Sprinkle them over the vegetables on the pan and toss to coat with seasonings. Bake in the oven for 25 minutes. Stir frequently until vegetables are soft and lightly browned and chickpeas are crisp, for about 20 to 25 minutes more. Season with more salt and black pepper to taste, top with the green onion before serving.

Lemon Garlic Roasted Bean Sprouts andCauliflower

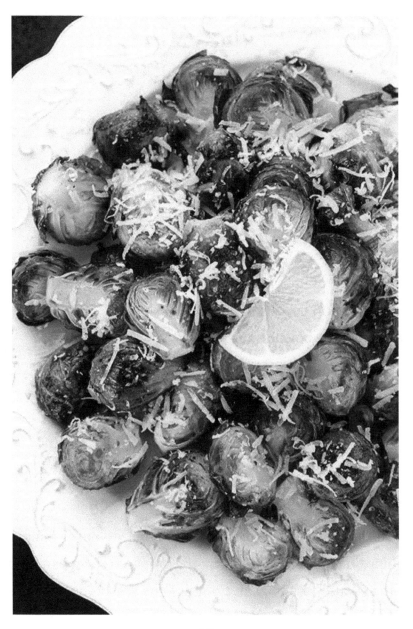

Ingredients

1 large cauliflower, sliced

1 cup bean sprouts

1 red onion, diced

1 potato, peeled and cut into 1-inch cubes

2 large carrots, cut into 1 inch pieces

3 medium potatoes, cut into 1-inch pieces

3 tablespoons melted vegan butter/ margarine

Seasoning Ingredients

1 teaspoon lemon

salt

1/2 teaspoonground black pepper

1 teaspoon onion powder

2 teaspoongarlic powder

Garnishing Ingredients

2 green onions, chopped (optional)

Directions:

Preheat your oven to 350 degrees F. Grease your baking pan. Combine the main Ingredients on the prepared sheet pan. Drizzle with the oil and toss to coat. Combine the seasoning Ingredients in a bowl Sprinkle them over the vegetables on the pan and toss to coat with seasonings. Bake in the oven for 25 minutes. Stir frequently until vegetables are soft and lightly browned and chickpeas are crisp, for about 20 to 25 minutes more. Season with more salt and black pepper to taste, top with the green onion before serving.

Roasted Broccoli Sweet Potatoes & Bean Sprouts

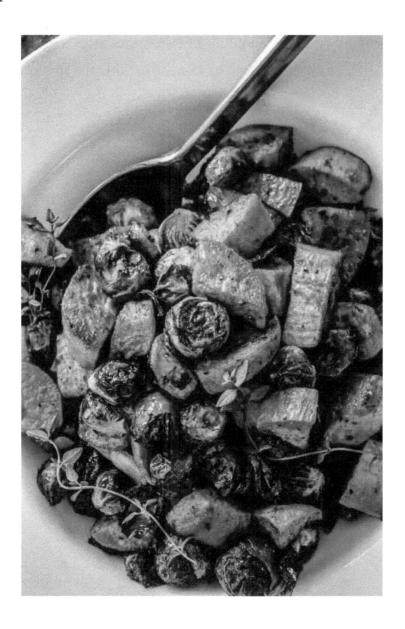

Ingredients

1 large broccoli, sliced

1 cup bean sprouts

1 yellow onion, diced

1 sweet potato, peeled and cut into 1-inch cubes

2 large carrots, cut into 1 inch pieces

3 medium potatoes, cut into 1-inch pieces

3 tablespoons canola oil

Seasoning Ingredients

1 teaspoon salt

1/2 teaspoonground black pepper

1 teaspoon onion powder

2 teaspoongarlic powder

½ cup grated gouda cheese

¼ cup parmesan cheese

Garnishing Ingredients

2 green onions, chopped (optional)

Directions:

Preheat your oven to 350 degrees F. Grease your baking pan. Combine the main Ingredients on the prepared sheet pan. Drizzle with the oil and toss to coat. Combine the seasoning Ingredients in a bowl Sprinkle them over the vegetables on the pan and toss to coat with seasonings. Bake in the oven for 25 minutes. Stir frequently until vegetables are soft and lightly browned and chickpeas are crisp, for about 20 to 25 minutes more. Season with more salt and black pepper to taste, top with the green onion before serving.

Baked Rainbow Carrots and Brussel Sprouts

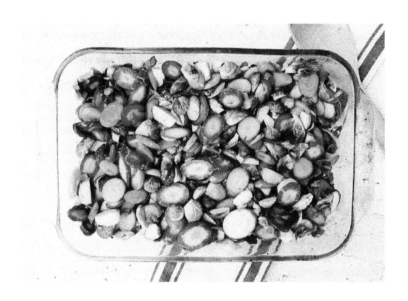

Ingredients

1 ½ cups Brussels sprouts, trimmed

1 cup large potato chunks

1 cup large rainbow carrot chunks

1 ½ cup broccoli florets

1 cup cubed red beets

1/2 cup red onion chunks

2 tablespoons extra-virgin olive oil

salt and ground black pepper to taste

Directions:

Preheat your oven to 425 degrees F (220 degrees C). Set the rack to the second-lowest level in the oven. Pour some lightly salted water in a bowl. Submerge the Brussels sprouts in salted water for 15 minutes and drain. Place the rest of the Ingredients together in a bowl. Spread the vegetables in a single layer onto a baking pan. Roast in the oven until the vegetables start to brown and cook through, for about 45 minutes.

Roasted Sweet Potato and Red Beets

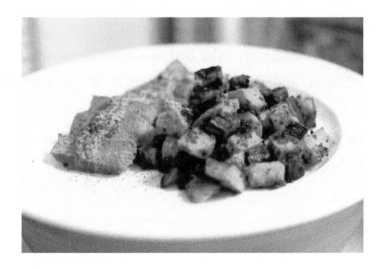

Ingredients

1 ½ cups Brussels sprouts, trimmed

1 cup large sweet potato chunks

1 cup large carrot chunks

1 ½ cup broccoli florets

salt and ground black pepper

1 cup cubed red beets

1/2 cup yellow onion chunks

2 tablespoons sesame seed oil

salt and ground black pepper to taste

Directions:

Preheat your oven to 425 degrees F (220 degrees C). Set the rack to the second-lowest level in the oven. Pour some lightly salted water in a bowl. Submerge the Brussels sprouts in salted water for 15 minutes and drain. Place the rest of the Ingredients together in a bowl. Spread the vegetables in a single layer onto a baking pan. Roast in the oven until the vegetables start to brown and cook through, for about 45 minutes.

Roasted Purple Cabbage and Beets

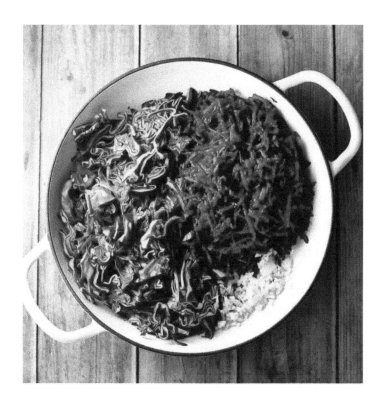

Ingredients

1 ½ cups purple cabbage, trimmed

1 cup large potato chunks

1 cup large carrot chunks

1 ½ cup cauliflower florets

1 cup cubed red beets

1/2 cup Vidalia onion chunks

2 tablespoons extra-virgin olive oil

Sea salt and ground black pepper to taste

Directions:

Preheat your oven to 425 degrees F (220 degrees C). Set the rack to the second-lowest level in the oven. Pour some lightly salted water in a bowl. Submerge the purple cabbage in salted water for 15 minutes and drain. Place the rest of the Ingredients together in a bowl. Spread the vegetables in a single layer onto a baking pan. Roast in the oven until the vegetables start to brown and cook through, for about 45 minutes.

Sichuan Style Baked Choggia Beets and Broccoli Florets

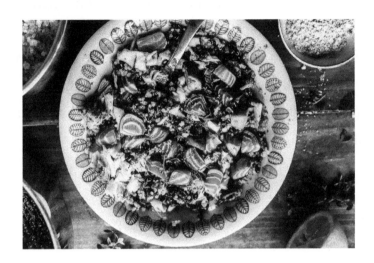

Ingredients

1 ½ cups Brussels sprouts, trimmed

1 cup broccoli florets

1 cup Choggia beets, cut into chunks

1 ½ cup cauliflower florets

1 cup button mushrooms, sliced

1/2 cup red onion chunks

2 tablespoons sesame oil

½ tsp. Sichuan peppercorns

salt ground black pepper to taste

Directions:

Preheat your oven to 425 degrees F (220 degrees C). Set the rack to the second-lowest level in the oven. Pour some lightly salted water in a bowl. Submerge the Brussels sprouts in salted water for 15 minutes and drain. Place the rest of the Ingredients together in a bowl. Spread the vegetables in a single layer onto a baking pan. Roast in the oven until the vegetables start to brown and cook through, for about 45 minutes.

Spicy and Smoky Baked Brussels Sprouts and Red Beets

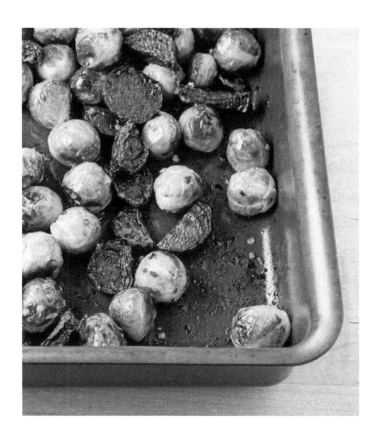

Ingredients

1 ½ cups Brussels sprouts, trimmed

1 cup large potato chunks

1 cup large red beets cut into chunks

1 ½ cup cauliflower florets

1 cup cubed red beets

1/2 cup red onion chunks

1 tsp. cumin

1 tsp. cayenne pepper

2 tablespoons extra-virgin olive oil

salt and ground black pepper to taste

Directions:

Preheat your oven to 425 degrees F (220 degrees C). Set the rack to the second-lowest level in the oven. Pour some lightly salted water in a bowl. Submerge the Brussels sprouts in salted water for 15 minutes and drain. Place the rest of the Ingredients together in a bowl. Spread the vegetables in a single layer onto a baking pan. Roast in the oven until the vegetables start to brown and cook through, for about 45 minutes.

Baked Enoki and Mini Cabbage

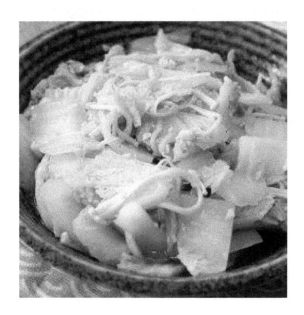

Ingredients

1 ½ cups mini cabbage, trimmed

1 cup broccoli florets

1 cup enoki mushrooms, sliced

1 ½ cup cauliflower florets

1 cup oyster mushrooms

1/2 cup red onion chunks

2 tablespoons olive oil

salt and ground black pepper to taste

Directions:

Preheat your oven to 425 degrees F (220 degrees C). Set the rack to the second-lowest level in the oven. Pour some lightly salted water in a bowl. Submerge the Brussels sprouts in salted water for 15 minutes and drain. Place the rest of the Ingredients together in a bowl. Spread the vegetables in a single layer onto a baking pan. Roast in the oven until the vegetables start to brown and cook through, for about 45 minutes.

Roasted Spinach Brussels Sprouts and Broccoli

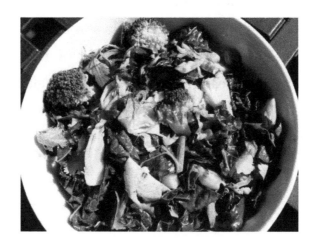

Ingredients

1 ½ cups Brussels sprouts, trimmed

1 cup spinach, coarsely chopped

1 cup romaine lettuce, coarsely chopped

1 ½ cup cauliflower florets

1 cup broccoli florets

1/2 cup red onion chunks

2 tablespoons extra-virgin olive oil

Sea salt and ground rainbow peppercorns to taste

¼ cup grated parmesan

Directions:

Preheat your oven to 425 degrees F (220 degrees C). Set the rack to the second-lowest level in the oven. Pour some lightly salted water in a bowl. Submerge the Brussels sprouts in salted water for 15 minutes and drain. Place the rest of the Ingredients together in a bowl. Spread the vegetables in a single layer onto a baking pan. Roast in the oven until the vegetables start to brown and cook through, for about 45 minutes.

Roasted Triple Mushrooms

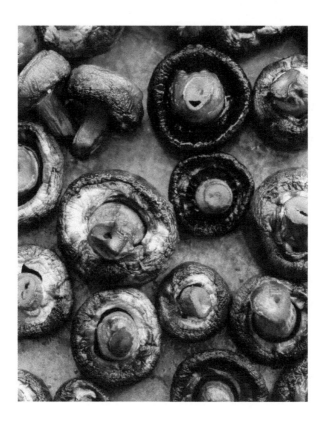

Ingredients

2 cups Spinach, rinsed

1 cup oyster mushrooms

1 cup button mushrooms, sliced

1 ½ cup enoki mushrooms

1/2 cup red onion chunks

2 tablespoons extra-virgin olive oil

salt and ground black pepper to taste

1/4 cup Ricotta cheese

Directions:

Preheat your oven to 425 degrees F (220 degrees C). Set the rack to the second-lowest level in the oven. Pour some lightly salted water in a bowl. Submerge the spinach in salted water for 15 minutes and drain. Place the rest of the Ingredients together in a bowl. Spread the vegetables in a single layer onto a baking pan. Roast in the oven until the vegetables start to brown and cook through, for about 45 minutes.

Roasted Mini Cabbage Rainbow Carrots & Bean Sprouts

Ingredients

1 ½ cups mini cabbage, trimmed

1 cup bean sprouts

1 cup large rainbow carrot chunks

1 ½ cup cauliflower florets

1 cup broccoli florets

1/2 cup red onion chunks

2 tablespoons canola oil

2 tbsp. Thai chili garlic paste

1 Thai basil

salt and ground black pepper to taste

Directions:

Preheat your oven to 425 degrees F (220 degrees C). Set the rack to the second-lowest level in the oven. Pour some lightly salted water in a bowl. Submerge the mini cabbage in salted water for 15 minutes and drain. Place the rest of the Ingredients together in a bowl. Spread the vegetables in a single layer onto a baking pan.

Roast in the oven until the vegetables start to brown and cook through, for about 45 minutes.

Roasted Mini Cabbage and Sweet Potato

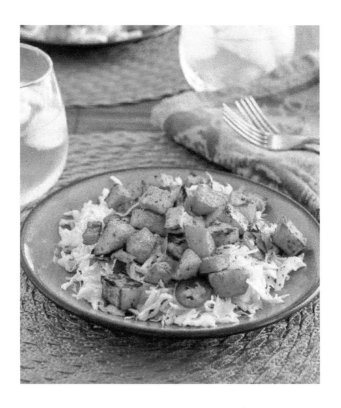

Ingredients

1 ½ cups mini cabbage, trimmed

1 cup large potato chunks

1 cup large rainbow carrot chunks

1 ½ cup potato chunks

1 cup parsnips

1/2 cup red onion chunks

2 tablespoons extra-virgin olive oil

Sea salt

Rainbow peppercorns to taste

1/4 cup cottage cheese

Directions:

Preheat your oven to 425 degrees F (220 degrees C). Set the rack to the second-lowest level in the oven. Pour some lightly salted water in a bowl. Submerge the mini cabbage in salted water for 15 minutes and drain. Place the rest of the Ingredients together in a bowl. Spread the vegetables in a single layer onto a baking pan. Roast in the oven until the vegetables start to brown and cook through, for about 45 minutes.

Roasted Buttery Brussels Sprouts & Cauliflower

Ingredients

1 ½ cups brussels sprouts, trimmed

1 cup large potato chunks

1 cup large carrot chunks

1 ½ cup cauliflower florets

1 cup sweet potato chunks

1/2 cup red onion chunks

2 tablespoons vegan butter/ margarine

Sea salt and ground black pepper to taste

Directions:

Preheat your oven to 425 degrees F (220 degrees C). Set the rack to the second-lowest level in the oven. Pour some lightly salted water in a bowl. Submerge the brussels sprouts in salted water for 15 minutes and drain. Place the rest of the Ingredients together in a bowl. Spread the vegetables in a single layer onto a baking pan. Roast in the oven until the vegetables start to brown and cook through, for about 45 minutes.

Roasted Red Potatoes and Asparagus

Ingredients

1 1/2 pounds red potatoes, cut into chunks

2 tablespoons extra virgin olive oil

12 cloves garlic, thinly sliced

1 tbsp. and 1 tsp. dried rosemary

4 teaspoons dried thyme

2 teaspoons sea salt

1 bunch fresh asparagus, trimmed and cut into 1 inch pieces

Directions:

Preheat your oven to 425 degrees F. In a baking pan, combine the first 5 Ingredients and 1/2 of the sea salt. Cover with foil. Bake 20 minutes in the oven. Combine the asparagus, oil, and salt. Cover, and cook for about 15 minutes, or until the potatoes becomes tender. Increase your oven temperature to 450 degrees F. Take out the foil, and cook for 8 minutes, until potatoes become lightly browned.

Baked Parsnips and Green Beans

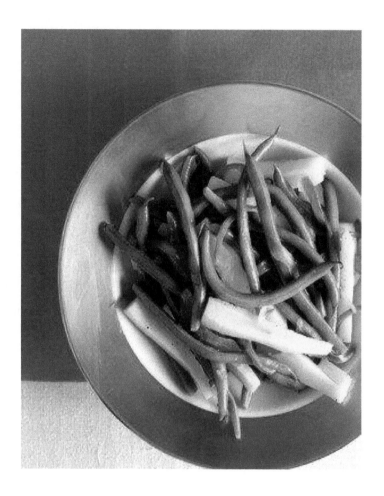

Ingredients

1 1/2 pounds parsnips, cut into chunks

2 tablespoons extra virgin olive oil

12 cloves garlic, thinly sliced

1 tbsp. and 1 tsp. Italian seasoning

4 teaspoons dried thyme

2 teaspoons sea salt

1 bunch green beans, trimmed and cut into 1 inch pieces

Directions:

Preheat your oven to 425 degrees F. In a baking pan, combine the first 5 Ingredients and 1/2 of the sea salt. Cover with foil. Bake 20 minutes in the oven. Combine the green beans, oil, and salt. Cover, and cook for about 15 minutes, or until the parsnips becomes tender. Increase your oven temperature to 450 degrees F. Take out the foil, and cook for 8 minutes, until potatoes become lightly browned.

Roasted Lime Garlic Buttered Green Beans

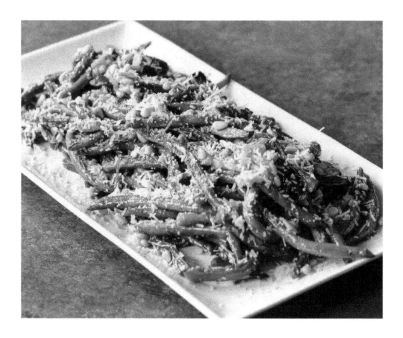

Ingredients

1 1/2 pounds potatoes, cut into chunks

4 tablespoons butter

12 cloves garlic, thinly sliced

2 tsp. lime juice

2 teaspoons sea salt

1 bunch fresh green beans, trimmed and cut into 1 inch pieces

Directions:

Preheat your oven to 425 degrees F. In a baking pan, combine the first 5 Ingredients and 1/2 of the sea salt. Cover with foil. Bake 20 minutes in the oven. Combine the green beans, oil, and salt. Cover, and cook for about 15 minutes, or until the potatoes becomes tender. Increase your oven temperature to 450 degrees F. Take out the foil, and cook for 8 minutes, until potatoes become lightly browned.

Roasted Parsnips and Edamame Beans

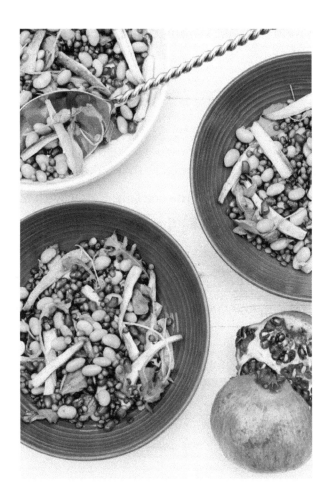

Ingredients

1 1/2 pounds parsnips, cut into chunks

2 tablespoons extra virgin olive oil

12 cloves garlic, thinly sliced

1 tbsp. dried rosemary

4 teaspoons dried thyme

2 teaspoons sea salt

1 bunch edamame beans , trimmed and cut into 1 inch pieces

Directions:

Preheat your oven to 425 degrees F. In a baking pan, combine the first 5 Ingredients and 1/2 of the sea salt. Cover with foil. Bake 20 minutes in the oven. Combine the edamame beans, oil, and salt. Cover, and cook for about 15 minutes, or until the turnips becomes tender. Increase your oven temperature to 450 degrees F. Take out the foil, and cook for 8 minutes, until potatoes become lightly browned.

Roasted Escarole and Hearts of Palm

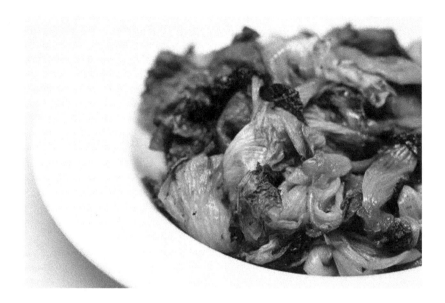

Ingredients

1 1/2 pounds escarole, cut into chunks

3 tablespoons extra virgin olive oil

12 cloves garlic, thinly sliced

1 tbsp. and 1 tsp. dried rosemary

4 teaspoons dried thyme

2 teaspoons sea salt

1 bunch hearts of palm, trimmed and cut into 1 inch pieces

Directions:

Preheat your oven to 425 degrees F. In a baking pan, combine the first 5 Ingredients and 1/2 of the sea salt. Cover with foil. Bake 20 minutes in the oven. Combine the hearts of palm, oil, and salt. Cover, and cook for about 15 minutes, or until the escarole becomes tender. Increase your oven temperature to 450 degrees F. Take out the foil, and cook for 8 minutes, until potatoes become lightly browned.

Roasted Lemon Green Beans and Red Potatoes

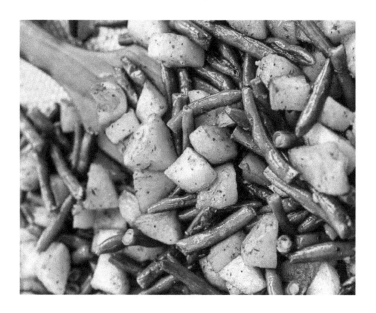

Ingredients

1 1/2 pounds red potatoes, cut into chunks

2 tablespoons salted butter

12 cloves garlic, thinly sliced

1 tbsp. lemon juice

1 tsp. annatto seeds

2 teaspoons sea salt

1 bunch green beans, trimmed and cut into 1 inch pieces

Directions:

Preheat your oven to 425 degrees F. In a baking pan, combine the first 5 Ingredients and 1/2 of the sea salt. Cover with foil. Bake 20 minutes in the oven. Combine the asparagus, oil, and salt. Cover, and cook for about 15 minutes, or until the potatoes becomes tender. Increase your oven temperature to 450 degrees F. Take out the foil, and cook for 8 minutes, until potatoes become lightly browned.

Roasted Italian Kohlrabi and Asparagus

Ingredients

1 1/2 pounds kohlrabi, cut into chunks

2 tablespoons extra virgin olive oil

12 cloves garlic, thinly sliced

1 tsp. Italian seasoning

4 teaspoons dried thyme

2 teaspoons sea salt

1 bunch fresh asparagus, trimmed and cut into 1 inch pieces

Directions:

Preheat your oven to 425 degrees F. In a baking pan, combine the first 5 Ingredients and 1/2 of the sea salt. Cover with foil. Bake 20 minutes in the oven. Combine the asparagus, oil, and salt. Cover, and cook for about 15 minutes, or until the kohlrabi becomes tender. Increase your oven temperature to 450 degrees F. Take out the foil, and cook for 8 minutes, until kohlrabi become lightly browned.

Roasted Yucca Root, Turnips & Carrots

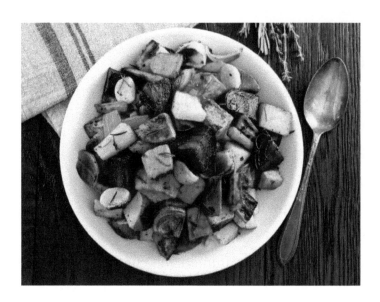

Ingredients

1/2 pound carrots, cut into chunks

½ pound yucca root, cut into chunks

½ pound turnips, cut into chunks

2 tablespoons extra virgin olive oil

12 cloves garlic, thinly sliced

1 tbsp. and 1 tsp. dried rosemary

4 teaspoons dried thyme

2 teaspoons sea salt

1 bunch fresh asparagus, trimmed and cut into 1 inch pieces

Directions:

Preheat your oven to 425 degrees F. In a baking pan, combine the first 7 Ingredients and 1/2 of the sea salt. Cover with foil. Bake 20 minutes in the oven. Combine the asparagus, oil, and salt. Cover, and cook for about 15 minutes, or until the root vegetables becomes tender. Increase your oven temperature to 450 degrees F. Take out the foil, and cook for 8 minutes, until yucca root become lightly browned.

Roasted Nutty Potato and Sweet Potato

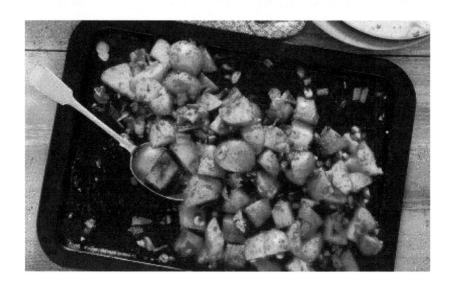

Ingredients

1/2 pounds red potatoes, cut into chunks

½ pound sweet potatoes, cut into chunks

2 tablespoons peanut oil

12 cloves garlic, thinly sliced

1 tbsp. and 1 tsp. herbs de Provence

2 teaspoons sea salt

1 bunch fresh asparagus, trimmed and cut into 1 inch pieces

Directions:

Preheat your oven to 425 degrees F. In a baking pan, combine the first 6 Ingredients and 1/2 of the sea salt. Cover with foil. Bake 20 minutes in the oven. Combine the asparagus, oil, and salt. Cover, and cook for about 15 minutes, or until the root vegetables becomes tender. Increase your oven temperature to 450 degrees F. Take out the foil, and cook for 8 minutes, until potatoes become lightly browned.

Roasted Yams and Asparagus

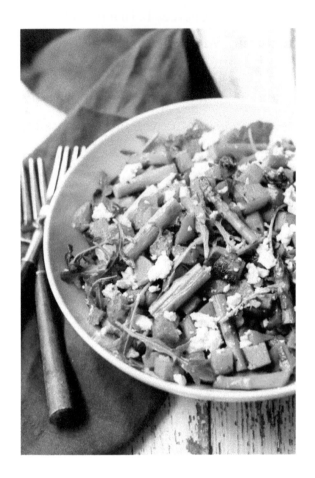

Ingredients

1/2 pound purple yam, cut into chunks

½ pound white yam, cut into chunks

½ pound sweet potato

2 tablespoons canola olive oil

12 cloves garlic, thinly sliced

2 tsp. Italian seasoning

2 teaspoons sea salt

1 bunch fresh asparagus, trimmed and cut into 1 inch pieces

Directions:

Preheat your oven to 425 degrees F. In a baking pan, combine the first 6 Ingredients and 1/2 of the sea salt. Cover with foil. Bake 20 minutes in the oven. Combine the asparagus, oil, and salt. Cover, and cook for about 15 minutes, or until the root vegetables becomes tender. Increase your oven temperature to 450 degrees F. Take out the foil, and cook for 8 minutes, until potatoes become lightly browned.

Baked Kohlrabi Yucca Root and Mustard Greens

Ingredients

1/2 pound kohlrabi, cut into chunks

½ pound yucca root, cut into chunks

½ pound mustard greens

2 tablespoons extra virgin olive oil

12 cloves garlic, thinly sliced

1 tbsp. and

1 tsp. dried rosemary

4 teaspoons dried thyme

2 teaspoons sea salt

1 bunch fresh green beans, trimmed and cut into 1 inch pieces

Directions:

Preheat your oven to 425 degrees F. In a baking pan, combine the first 7 Ingredients and 1/2 of the sea salt. Cover with foil. Bake 20 minutes in the oven. Combine the green beans, olive oil, and salt. Cover, and cook for about 15 minutes, or until the root vegetables becomes tender. Increase your oven temperature to 450 degrees

F. Take out the foil, and cook for 8 minutes, until potatoes become lightly browned.

Baked Brussel Sprouts & Red Onion Glazed with Balsamic Vinegar

Ingredients

1 (16 ounce) package fresh Brussels sprouts

2 small red onions, thinly sliced

¼ cup and 1 tbsp. extra-virgin olive oil, divided

1/4 teaspoon sea salt

1/4 teaspoon rainbow peppercorns

1 shallot, chopped

1/4 cup balsamic vinegar

1 tablespoon chopped fresh rosemary

Directions:

Preheat your oven to 425 degrees F (220 degrees C). Grease a baking pan. Combine Brussels sprouts and onion in a bowl Add 4 tablespoons olive oil, salt, and peppercorns Toss to coat and spread the sprouts mixture on the pan. Bake in the oven until sprouts and red onion become tender, for about 25 to 30 minutes. Heat the remaining tablespoon of olive oil in a small skillet over medium-high heat Sauté the shallots until tender, for about 5 minutes. Add balsamic vinegar and cook until the glaze is reduced for about 5 minutes. Add rosemary into the balsamic glaze and pour over the sprouts.

Baked Purple Cabbage with Rainbow Peppercorns

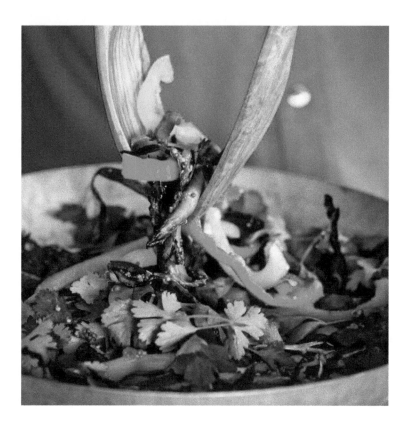

Ingredients

1 (16 ounce) package fresh purple cabbage

2 small red onions, thinly sliced

1/2 cup and 1 tbsp. extra-virgin olive oil, divided

1/4 teaspoon sea salt

1/4 teaspoon rainbow peppercorns

1 shallot, chopped

1/4 cup balsamic vinegar

1 tsp. herbs de Provence

Directions:

Preheat your oven to 425 degrees F (220 degrees C). Grease a baking pan. Combine cabbage and onion in a bowl Add 4 tablespoons olive oil, salt, and peppercorns Toss to coat and spread the sprouts mixture on the pan. Bake in the oven until sprouts and onion become tender, for about 25 to 30 minutes. Heat the remaining tablespoon of olive oil in a small skillet over medium-high heat Sauté the shallots until tender, for about 5 minutes. Add balsamic vinegar and cook until the glaze is reduced for about 5 minutes. Add herbs de Provence into the balsamic glaze and pour over the sprouts.

Roasted Savoy Cabbage and Vidalia Onion

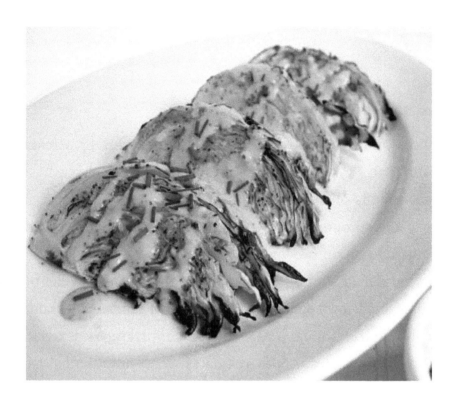

Ingredients

1 (16 ounce) package fresh Savoy Cabbage

2 Vidalia onions, thinly sliced

¼ cup and 1 tbsp. extra-virgin olive oil, divided

1/4 teaspoon sea salt

1/4 teaspoon black peppercorns

1 shallot, chopped

1/4 cup white wine vinegar

1 tablespoon chopped fresh rosemary

Directions:

Preheat your oven to 425 degrees F (220 degrees C). Grease a baking pan. Combine cabbage and onion in a bowl Add 4 tablespoons olive oil, salt, and peppercorns Toss to coat and spread the sprouts mixture on the pan. Bake in the oven until sprouts and onion become tender, for about 25 to 30 minutes. Heat the remaining tablespoon of olive oil in a small skillet over medium-high heat Sauté the shallots until tender, for about 5 minutes. Add white wine vinegar and cook until the glaze is reduced for about 5 minutes. Add rosemary into the balsamic glaze and pour over the sprouts.

Baked Crimini Mushrooms and Red Potatoes

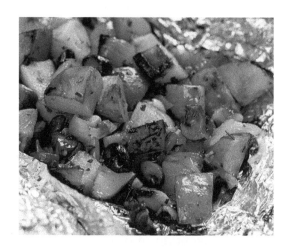

Ingredients

1 pound red potatoes, halved

2 tablespoons extra virgin olive oil

1/2 pound Cremini mushrooms

8 cloves unpeeled garlic

2 tablespoons chopped fresh thyme

1 tablespoon extra-virgin olive oil sea

salt and ground black pepper to taste

1/4 pound cherry tomatoes

3 tablespoons toasted pine nuts

1/4 pound spinach, thinly sliced

Directions:

Preheat your oven to 425 degrees F. Spread the potatoes in a pan Drizzle with 2 tablespoons of olive oil and roast for 15 minutes turning once. Add the mushrooms with the stem sides up Add the garlic cloves to pan and cook until lightly browned Sprinkle with thyme. Drizzle with 1 tablespoon olive oil and season with sea salt and black pepper. Return to the oven and bake for 5 min. Add the cherry tomatoes to the pan. Return to oven and bake until mushrooms become softened, for 5 min. Sprinkle the pine nuts over the potatoes and mushrooms. Serve with the spinach.

Baked Shitake Mushrooms and Kohlrabi

Ingredients

1 pound kohlrabi, halved

2 tablespoons extra virgin olive oil

1/2 pound shitake mushrooms

8 cloves unpeeled garlic

3 tablespoons sesame oil sea

salt and ground black pepper to taste

1/4 pound cherry tomatoes

3 tablespoons toasted cashew nuts

1/4 pound spinach, thinly sliced

Directions:

Spread the potatoes in a pan Drizzle with 2 tablespoons of oil and Preheat your oven to 425 degrees F. roast for 15 minutes turning once. Add the mushrooms with the stem sides up Add the garlic cloves to pan and cook until lightly browned Drizzle with 1 tablespoon sesame oil and season with sea salt and black pepper. Return to the oven and bake for 5 min. Add the cherry tomatoes to the pan. Return to oven and bake until mushrooms become softened, for 5 min. Sprinkle the cashew nuts over the kohlrabi and mushrooms. Serve with the spinach.

Baked Button Mushroom and Summer Squash

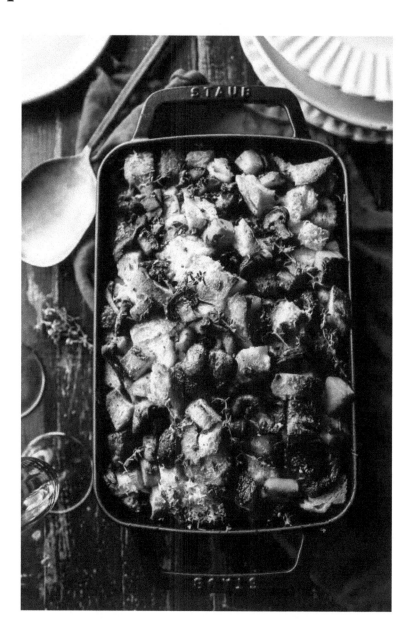

Ingredients

1 pound summer squash, halved

2 tablespoons extra virgin olive oil

1/2 pound button mushrooms

8 cloves unpeeled garlic

2 tsp. cumin

1 tsp. annatto seed

½ tsp. cayenne pepper

1 tablespoon extra-virgin olive oil sea

salt and ground black pepper to taste

1/4 pound cherry tomatoes

3 tablespoons toasted pine nuts

1/4 pound spinach, thinly sliced

Directions:

Preheat your oven to 425 degrees F. Spread the summer squash in a pan Drizzle with 2 tablespoons of olive oil and roast for 15 minutes turning once. Add the mushrooms with the stem sides up Add the garlic cloves to pan and cook until lightly browned Sprinkle with cumin, cayenne pepper and annatto seeds. Drizzle with 1 tablespoon olive oil and season with sea salt and black pepper. Return to the oven and bake for 5 min. Add the cherry tomatoes to the pan. Return to oven and bake until mushrooms become softened, for 5 min. Sprinkle the pine nuts over the summer squash and mushrooms. Serve with the spinach.

Baked Spinach and Butternut Squash

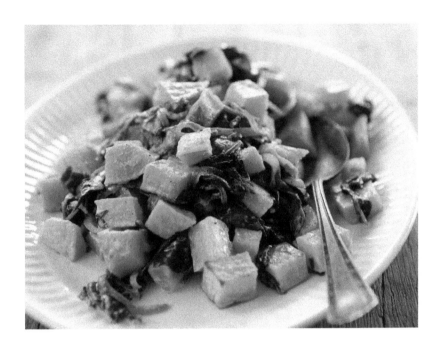

Ingredients

1 ½ pounds butternut squash, peeled and cut into 1-inch chunks

½ red onion, thinly sliced

¼ cup water

½ vegetable stock cube, crumbled

1 tbsp. extra virgin olive oil

½ tsp cumin

½ tsp annatto seeds

½ tsp cayenne pepper

½ tsp hot chili powder

Black pepper

½ pound fresh spinach, roughly chopped

Directions:

Put all of the Ingredients in a slow cooker except the last one. Top with handfuls of spinach and stuff the slow cooker with it. If you can't fit it all in at once, let the first batch cook first and add some more spinach. Cook for 3or 4 hours on medium until squash become soft. Scrape the sides and serve.

Baked Watercress and Summer Squash

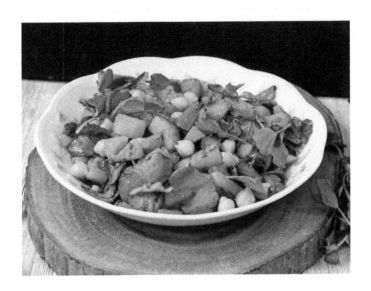

Ingredients

1 ½ pounds summer squash, peeled and cut into 1-inch chunks

½ red onion, thinly sliced

¼ cup water

½ vegetable stock cube, crumbled

1 tbsp. sesame oil

½ tsp Chinese

5 spice powder

½ tsp Sichuan Peppercorns

½ tsp hot chili powder

Black pepper

½ pound fresh watercress, roughly chopped

Directions:

Put all of the Ingredients in a slow cooker except the last one. Top with handfuls of watercress and stuff the slow cooker with it. If you can't fit it all in at once, let the first batch cook first and add some more watercress. Cook for 3 or 4 hours on medium until summer squash become soft. Scrape the sides and serve.

Curried Kale and Rutabaga

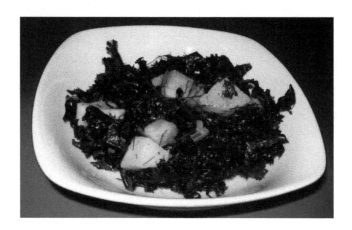

Ingredients

1 ½ pounds Rutabaga, peeled and cut into 1-inch chunks

½ onion, thinly sliced

¼ cup water

½ vegetable stock cube, crumbled

1 tbsp. extra virgin olive oil

½ tsp cumin

½ tsp ground coriander

½ tsp garam masala

½ tsp hot chili powder

Black pepper

½ pound fresh kale, roughly chopped

Directions:

Put all of the Ingredients in a slow cooker except the last one. Top with handfuls of kale and stuff the slow cooker with it. If you can't fit it all in at once, let the first batch cook first and add some more kale. Cook for 3or 4 hours on medium until root vegetables become soft. Scrape the sides and serve.

Buttered Potatoes and Spinach

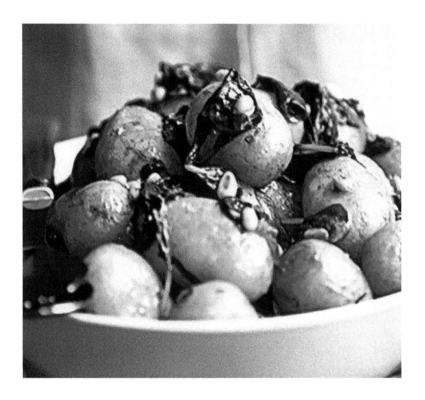

Ingredients

1 ½ pounds red potatoes, peeled and cut into 1-inch chunks

½ onion, thinly sliced

¼ cup water

½ vegetable stock cube, crumbled

2 tbsp. salted butter

½ tsp herbs de Provence

½ tsp thyme

½ tsp hot chili powder

Black pepper

½ pound fresh spinach, roughly chopped

Directions:

Put all of the Ingredients in a slow cooker except the last one. Top with handfuls of spinach and stuff the slow cooker with it. If you can't fit it all in at once, let the first batch cook first and add some more spinach. Cook for 3or 4 hours on medium until potatoes become soft. Scrape the sides and serve.

Roasted Vegan-Buttered Mustard Greens Carrots

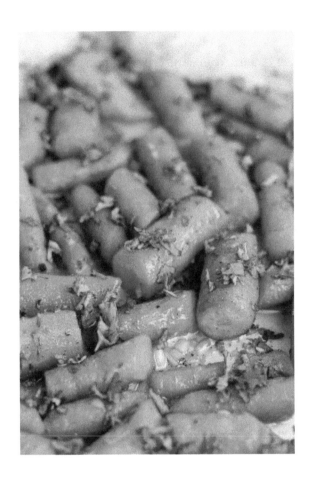

Ingredients

1 ½ pounds carrots, peeled and cut into 1-inch chunks

½ onion, thinly sliced

¼ cup water

½ vegetable stock cube, crumbled

1 tbsp. butter

1 tsp garlic, minced

½ tsp lemon juice

Black pepper

½ pound fresh mustard greens, roughly chopped

Directions:

Put all of the Ingredients in a slow cooker except the last one. Top with handfuls of mustard greens and stuff the slow cooker with it. If you can't fit it all in at once, let the first batch cook first and add some more mustard greens. Cook for 3or 4 hours on medium until carrots become soft. Scrape the sides and serve.

Smoky Roasted Swiss Chard and Cauliflower

Ingredients

1 ½ pounds cauliflower, peeled and cut into 1-inch chunks

½ red onion, thinly sliced

¼ cup water

½ vegetable stock cube, crumbled

1 tbsp. extra virgin olive oil

½ tsp cumin

½ tsp hot chili powder

Black pepper

½ pound fresh Swiss chard, roughly chopped

Directions:

Put all of the Ingredients in a slow cooker except the last one. Top with handfuls of Swiss chard and stuff the slow cooker with it. If you can't fit it all in at once, let the first batch cook first and add some more Swiss chard. Cook for 3or 4 hours on medium until potatoes become soft. Scrape the sides and serve.

Roasted Microgreens and Potatoes

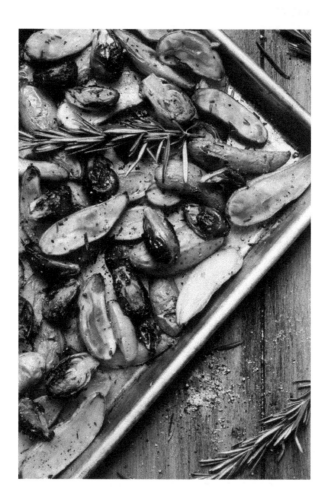

Ingredients

1 ½ pounds potatoes, peeled and cut into 1-inch chunks

½ onion, thinly sliced

¼ cup water

½ vegetable stock cube, crumbled

1 tbsp. olive oil

½ tsp minced ginger

2 sprigs lemon grass

½ tsp green onions, minced

½ tsp hot chili powder

Black pepper

½ pound Microgreens, roughly chopped

Directions:

Put all of the Ingredients in a slow cooker except the last one. Top with handfuls of Microgreens and stuff the slow cooker with it. If you can't fit it all in at once, let the first batch cook first and add some more Microgreens. Cook for 3or 4 hours on medium until potatoes become soft. Scrape the sides and serve.

Roasted Spinach & Broccoli with Jalapeno

Ingredients

1 ½ pounds broccoli florets

½ onion, thinly sliced

¼ cup water

½ vegetable stock cube, crumbled

1 tbsp. extra virgin olive oil

½ tsp cumin

8 jalapeno peppers, finely chopped

1 ancho chili

½ tsp hot chili powder

Black pepper

½ pound fresh spinach, roughly chopped

Directions:

Put all of the Ingredients in a slow cooker except the last one. Top with handfuls of spinach and stuff the slow cooker with it. If you can't fit it all in at once, let the first batch cook first and add some more spinach. Cook for 3or 4 hours on medium until broccoli become soft. Scrape the sides and serve.

Spicy Baked Swiss Chard and Cauliflower

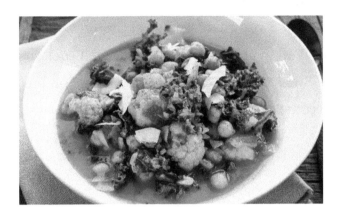

Ingredients

1 ½ pounds cauliflower florets, blanched (dipped in boiling water then dipped in ice water)

½ cup bean sprouts, rinsed

½ cup water

½ vegetable stock cube, crumbled

1 tbsp. sesame oil

½ tsp Thai chili paste

½ tsp Sriracha hot sauce

½ tsp hot chili powder

2 Thai bird chilies, minced

Black pepper

½ pound fresh Swiss chard, roughly chopped

Directions:

Put all of the Ingredients in a slow cooker except the last one. Top with handfuls of Swiss chard and stuff the slow cooker with it. If you can't fit it all in at once, let the first batch cook first and add some more Swiss chard. Cook for 3 or 4 hours on medium until potatoes become soft. Scrape the sides and serve.

Thai Carrots and Collard Greens

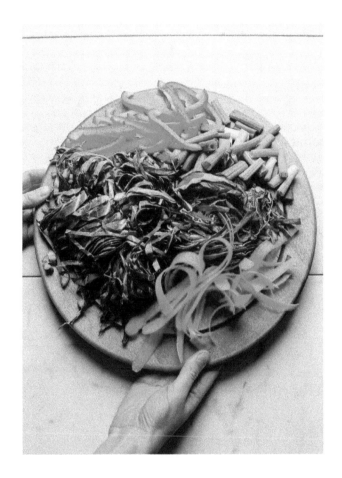

Ingredients

1 ½ pounds carrots, peeled and cut into 1-inch chunks

½ onion, thinly sliced

¼ cup water

½ vegetable stock cube, crumbled

1 tbsp. extra virgin olive oil

1 tbsp. sesame oil

½ tsp Thai chili paste

½ tsp Sriracha hot sauce

½ tsp hot chili powder

2 Thai bird chilies, minced

Black pepper

½ pound collard greens, roughly chopped

Directions:

Put all of the Ingredients in a slow cooker except the last one. Top with handfuls of collard greens and stuff the slow cooker with it. If you can't fit it all in at once, let the first batch cook first and add some more collard greens. Cook for 3or 4 hours on medium until carrots become soft. Scrape the sides and serve.

Baked White Yam and Spinach

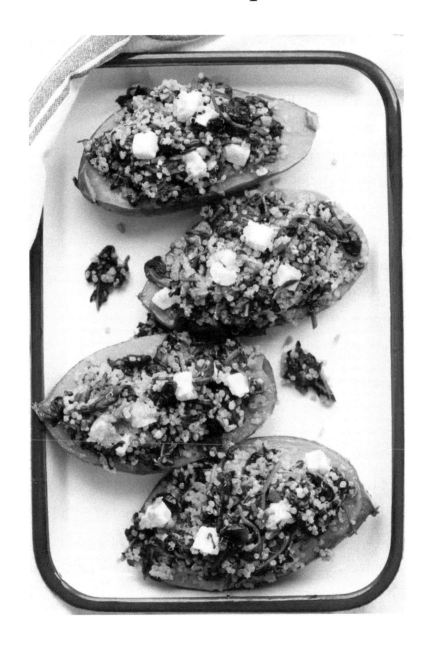

Ingredients

½ pounds potatoes, peeled and cut into 1-inch chunks

½ pounds white yam, peeled and cut into 1-inch chunks

½ pounds carrots, peeled and cut into 1-inch chunks

½ red onion, thinly sliced

¼ cup water

½ vegetable stock cube, crumbled

1 tbsp. extra virgin olive oil

½ tsp cumin

½ tsp ground coriander

½ tsp garam masala

½ tsp cayenne pepper

Black pepper

½ pound fresh spinach, roughly chopped

Directions:

Put all of the Ingredients in a slow cooker except the last one. Top with handfuls of spinach and stuff the slow cooker with it. If you can't fit it all in at once, let the first batch cook first and add some more spinach. Cook for 3or 4 hours on medium until potatoes become soft. Scrape the sides and serve.

Southeast Asian Baked Turnip Greens & Carrots

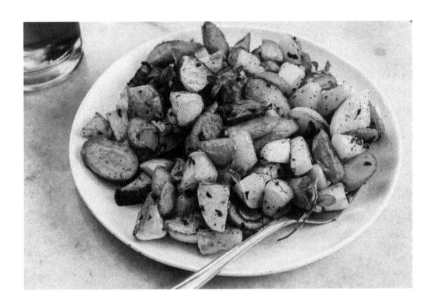

Ingredients

½ pound turnips, peeled and cut into 1-inch chunks

½ pound carrots, peeled and cut into 1-inch chunks

½ pound parsnips, peeled and cut into 1-inch chunks

½ red onion, thinly sliced

½ cup vegetable broth

1 tbsp. extra virgin olive oil

½ tsp minced ginger

2 stalks lemon grass

8 cloves garlic, minced

Black pepper

½ pound fresh turnip greens, roughly chopped

Directions:

Put all of the Ingredients in a slow cooker except the last one. Top with handfuls of turnip greens and stuff the slow cooker with it. If you can't fit it all in at once, let the first batch cook first and add some more turnip greens. Cook for 3or 4 hours on medium until turnips become soft. Scrape the sides and serve.

Curried Watercress and Potatoes

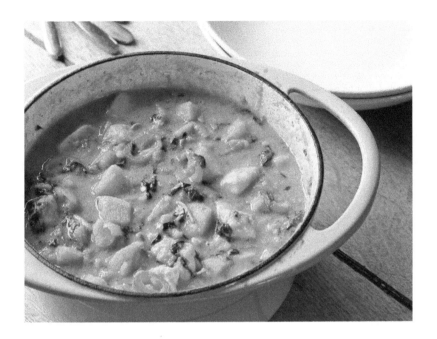

Ingredients

1 ½ pounds potatoes, peeled and cut into 1-inch chunks

½ onion, thinly sliced

¼ cup water

½ vegetable stock cube, crumbled

1 tbsp. extra virgin olive oil

½ tsp cumin

½ tsp ground coriander

½ tsp garam masala

½ tsp hot chili powder

Black pepper

½ pound fresh Watercress, roughly chopped

Directions:

Put all of the Ingredients in a slow cooker except the last one. Top with handfuls of watercress and stuff the slow cooker with it. If you can't fit it all in at once, let the first batch cook first and add some more watercress. Cook for 3or 4 hours on medium until potatoes become soft. Scrape the sides and serve.

Jalapeno Kale and Parsnips

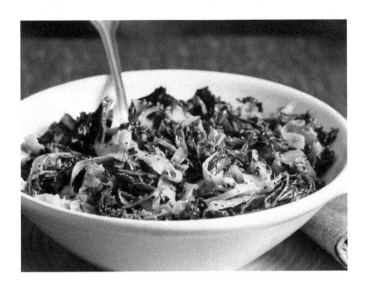

Ingredients

1 ½ pounds parsnips, peeled and cut into 1-inch chunks

½ red onion, thinly sliced

¼ cup water

½ vegetable stock cube, crumbled

1 tbsp. extra virgin olive oil

½ tsp cumin

½ tsp jalapeno pepper, minced

1 ancho chili, minced

Black pepper

½ pound Kale, roughly chopped

Directions:

Put all of the Ingredients in a slow cooker except the last one. Top with handfuls of kale and stuff the slow cooker with it. If you can't fit it all in at once, let the first batch cook first and add some more Kale. Cook for 3or 4 hours on medium until parsnips become soft. Scrape the sides and serve.

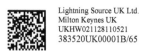